Speaking My TRUTH

Abdulahi Hassan

◆ FriesenPress

One Printers Way
Altona, MB R0G 0B0
Canada

www.friesenpress.com

Foreword by Jim Carr

ISBN
978-1-03-915891-7 (Hardcover)
978-1-03-915890-0 (Paperback)
978-1-03-915892-4 (eBook)

1. BIOGRAPHY & AUTOBIOGRAPHY, PERSONAL MEMOIRS

Distributed to the trade by The Ingram Book Company

FOREWORD

HELLO, MY NAME IS Jim Carr, and I am the head coordinator and professor of the Broadcasting –Radio diploma program at Seneca College (not the politician from Winnipeg), where I have been teaching for about twenty-five years. I try to give my students the tools to aid them in a plethora of production pathways, including: radio commercials, public service announcements and fifteen-second station identification spots. My goal is to watch my students become successful in every aspect of the program.

By the time Abdi Hassan rolled into my life, I'd already had a pretty big handful of students of his type: those who were often told "*no,*" who didn't learn like most, and were often overlooked; the students with mental or physical challenges that put them in special classes with support workers and lots of trips to the museum and to the zoo; the students in overworked education systems' who have a "*once in a lifetime challenge*" every single day of their lives.

Steve is blind, Beth is missing an arm, Dave is in a wheelchair, Fred is on one end of the spectrum, while Denise is on the other. Yes, I have learned and cared and figured out what has to happen to teach for success in any situation and it does require lots of time, effort, and quiet, often painting outside of the lines that frame "normal education," but the reward is far greater than any "regular student," and it was Abdi who taught me this.

I remember once in the middle of one of my classes, watching a student get up from their chair and walk across the room to tie Abdi's shoe because they noticed it was undone. That kind of compassion and caring only comes from having an Abdi in your class. I think the biggest cheer in his first semester production class came after the class watched Abdi, with hope and amazement, do an in-class exercise for the first time. It was a basic task and really not that big of a deal, but with the classes' perception of his ability already caught up in the big wheels of his motorized throne and the focus required to simply move the little stick to allow him to navigate the halls, it looked like the most challenging operation in the world.

During the time Abdi was a student, I had some personal struggles in my life, which have continued after he graduated. But when I wake up to an encouraging text message from Abdi such as: *Shine a beautiful light on yourself anytime you feel down or discouraged about anything going on in your life. It doesn't hurt to have a little bit of self-love once in a while* or *Just wanted to let you know I appreciate you so much for being you*, it is like my life has been infected by the best ever spam message virus, and when I don't even know I need it, I receive an echoed life lesson, showing me that things are going to be okay.

What is the measure of one's life in biography terms? Is it two pages, a thousand words, or a trillion syllables? The truth is, it is what tells the truth of one's life and for Abdi, that truth is one thing— hope... and *Speaking My Truth* screams hope from the tallest mountain. I will never forget the difference this amazing man has made in my life.

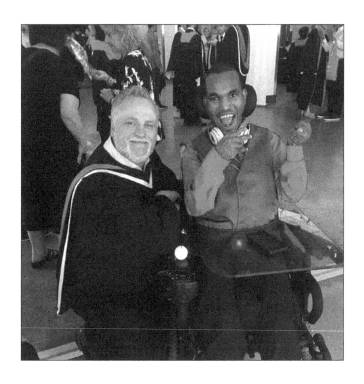

CHAPTER 1:

Welcome to the World of Abdi

MY NAME IS ABDULAHI Hassan—but most of my peers call me Abdi. I am a twenty-six-year-old Somali-Muslim man from Toronto, Ontario, Canada, living with a physical disability called cerebral palsy, which requires me to use a power wheelchair. Now before I go on with my story, I should explain what cerebral palsy is. Cerebral palsy is defined as a group of disorders that affect a person's ability to move and maintain balance and posture (CDC).

I was born three months premature, on May 30, 1996, at Humber River Hospital in North York, Ontario. The doctors didn't know if I would survive, and if I did, what long-term health issues I would have or what my capabilities would be. Some of the doctors' concerns included whether I would be able to speak, walk, or ultimately, even survive, which thankfully, I did.

Prior to going to school, it felt like I was the only person with cerebral palsy because I had never met anyone else like me. I also dealt with lots of physical pain on a daily basis, and although today I try to view every challenge in my life with a positive mindset, this wasn't always the case.

When I was younger, I often let people speak up for me, whether it was family members or teachers. For example, if I went to the mall to get a haircut, and I wanted to grab something to eat after, I would get my mom or whoever was with me to order for me, despite knowing that I was capable of doing it myself. Looking back, this stemmed from a fear of trying to build independence. Since I was so comfortable with it, I continued to use this method well into my teens, my early twenties, and sometimes until this day, depending on the situation.

In elementary school, I was always a funny, out-going, charming individual. This was also a point of deeper self-discovery, where I learned that I was a bad driver. My first taste of independence was moving from being pushed around in a regular wheelchair to a power wheelchair that I had full control over. I thought it would be easy to navigate, but I soon realized that wasn't the case. I remember attaching myself to my teachers, educational assistants, and other staff members, getting them to do things that I knew I was capable of doing, as I was scared of being independent. For instance, I had someone stand in line to buy my lunch. That was something that kind of scared me because of the amount of people that were in line, and I was scared of getting yelled at and feeling discouraged.

Another example of realizing my fear of independence was during the eighth grade, which was my last year of elementary school. I was very worried about what high school I was going to attend in the fall and the reality of being in a new in environment and not being able to enjoy my farewell elementary school tour. But we live and we learn.

Fast-forward to high school. It was a place where, as each year went by, I learned more and more about who I was as a person. Being able to speak up for myself was new to me, like when I told my high school guidance counsellor that I wanted to do co-op, which I will speak about later on this journey of mine.

I have a wonderful family, consisting of my mother Habibo, myself, and my four siblings: my eldest brother Mohammed—followed by me—my two younger sisters Hamdi and Shukri, and my youngest brother Abdikarim. At the time of this writing, we all live at home with our mom. Our father passed away, but I'll get into that later.

I'll start with the queen of all queens and no, I'm not talking about the queen of England. I'm talking about my mother, who is royalty in her own right. She is one of the strongest, most beautiful, and funny—so funny that I laugh before I can even retell her jokes—people I know. It blows my mind that she was able to raise the five of us while working as a school bus driver, then still come home after a long day on the road and cook, clean, etc.

I always pray for my mom because she is my biggest blessing/supporter. Once during Ramadan, which is the month of forgiveness and fasting from sunrise to sunset, my mom and my little brother took a trip to one of the holiest places in the world, Makkah, Saudi Arabia. They performed Umrah, which is an Islamic pilgrimage journey. During this time, they visited the Holy Mosque and did night prayers and more importantly, they sought God's forgiveness and prayed for loved ones who had passed away, and in general. I remember her saying that while she was over there, she was going to pray to God that my memoir would be successful and blessed. I have so many wonderful memories of my mom but that one always comes to mind when I think of her. I hope that as I get older, I'll be able to take care of her because of all she has done for me and my siblings over the years.

I look forward to many more good times with my mom, and she did say that we are going to go to Africa together, where she is going to try to get me married. I was very hesitant for a long time, but now I'm surprisingly open to the idea. As they say, after God, a mother always knows best.

FYI, no matter how many years go by in my lifetime, I will always be a momma's boy. I hope she feels the same adoration toward me. If not, I'll move to New York instead and write a Broadway play about how much I love her. Kidding aside, I love my, Mom.

Mohammed is very mellow, and he is my go-to guy when I need anything in any capacity, like if

I need assistance to use the washroom or to be turned to my side so I can watch TV. I am grateful for what he does for me and how he has stepped up over the last few years, especially when my father became sick. Yes, we do butt heads, and I can admit to being a hothead sometimes. However, as much as I don't say it to him very often, I do love my brother very much.

My sister Hamdi, is one of the smartest people I know... and one of the most tenacious at that, but I'm too scared to say that to her face. She recently became a nurse, and it's safe to say that we all expected nothing but greatness from her. She hasn't done the Heimlich maneuver on any of us yet, but I know she knows what she is doing. Who really needs a doctor when I have my sister? Scratch that, I might still need a doctor, but my sister is a great start. Did I forget to mention that Hamdi is also a Toronto Raptors fan? Trust me, you do not want to mess with her when a Raptors game is on, especially when it is a close game. Hamdi is also the person I rely on when I need food; she's basically my Uber Eats driver. I love her dearly.

Shukri is the most determined, no-nonsense, self-driven person I know, and she can do anything if she sets her mind to it. I remember when she wanted to go on a trip to San Diego with her friends, but she was nervous because she had never been on an airplane before. She was so determined to go on that trip, and she didn't let anything stop her from that goal, even if it meant taking risks along the way. Shukri is also always there when I need her to do something for me, and we joke around a lot. I do annoy her very much, but I hope she knows that I appreciate everything she does for me (I guess she does now!).

Abdikarim, though the youngest, is actually the tallest person in our entire family, and he loves playing video games while yelling at the top of his lungs. It can be very irritating because you never know who he is hollering at or why, but the passion he has for gaming is unique.

He has really stepped up in terms of helping me with my needs. When Mohammed is absent, Abdikarim surprisingly fills those gaps of assistance. Even though I was very hesitant because he is only eighteen years old, he has proven that he is capable of taking care of me in emergency circumstances.

My father's name was Hussein, but most of his peers called him Burgal as a nickname. He worked hard for more than fifteen years at Toronto Pearson Airport until a back injury required him to leave his job.

Sadly, he passed away in 2020—which was one of the hardest days of my life. I will get into that a little later though, as I explain my journey in more depth. For now, just sit back and relax... but don't get too comfortable because in my world, it's always a bumpy ride (pun intended).

CHAPTER 2:

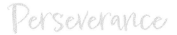

Perseverance

YOU NEVER KNOW WHAT'S going to happen in life, and for me, expecting the unexpected has been challenging but also very interesting. In 2011, I was diagnosed with type 1 diabetes, and to be honest, my first reaction was, "Wow, thank God it wasn't anything worse," but I also knew it would be difficult. I had been dealing with a whole host of other minor setbacks, including being underweight for my age, and these symptoms eventually led to the diagnosis of the diabetes. The doctors told me that I needed to check my blood sugar levels on a daily basis and take insulin. Being a fourteen-year-old kid, I treated it like it was nothing. I should have taken it more seriously, but I just wanted to feel normal. I wanted to live my life without constantly being reminded of my diabetes because the consequences from it scared me straight. But I continued to smile and take it with a grain of salt. I knew that it wouldn't be easy, but I just went with the flow.

I think the moment I realized my diabetes was holding me back in certain ways, was when I asked if I could do co-op. Co-operative education is designed for youth, around grade eleven or twelve, to gain experience in the workplace. I was assigned to work with an occupational therapist who gave people with disabilities a co-op placement. Before starting, I remember having a meeting with my mom, guidance counsellor, and the principal, as some administrators had expressed concerns about allowing me to do this co-op because of my diabetes. I later learned it was due to the fact that if my blood sugar was over ten, I couldn't go to my placement. It would have been nice if they had been transparent when it was actually happening. Granted, I was a sixteen-year-old at the time, but I would have had more respect for the decision-makers if they had the courtesy to tell me instead of me having to find out years later. At the time, their haste and inconsideration made me feel like I had no control over my independence and autonomy, which caused me to shift the blame to my diabetes diagnosis.

Thank God that one of my high school staff members advocated for me to be allowed to do the co-op placement. Some days were far more challenging than others, but being able to experience working in my community was really something else. Integrating was something new to me, and so was taking the bus on my own for the first time. But I knew those situations were going to get easier to deal with over time.

I learned a lot about working, and more importantly, about myself, during this time. One really cool thing I found out was that I was the first physically disabled student in my high school to do a co-op placement, which was a distinct honour that I will never forget.

I hope to work full-time in the future, however, at times, I feel discouraged to put myself out there because of my physical barriers. For example, my body gets stiff sometimes, which makes it difficult to navigate my wheelchair. I've learned that I have nothing to be ashamed of though, and no matter what happens, to keep pushing through and breaking boundaries for people like me.

The reason why I want to help individuals with disabilities to understand their potential is because back in high school, I had a teacher who actually questioned my abilities in front of my whole class, embarrassing me for not being able to colour properly. As an eighteen-year-old, I was speechless because I had never heard that before,... from any teacher of mine throughout my years of schooling, and it was done publicly to shame me. In the moment, everything felt numb. It was like a big punch in the gut. Furthermore, I felt like crying, but I somehow managed to keep it together. I did not respond to her comment. But looking back on it now, I laugh about it and remember how far I've come. I should have been proud of myself, no matter what that teacher said. Since then, I've learned that the only opinion that should matter to me is my own. Even if that teacher didn't realize that she hurt me, I still forgive her. As Muslims, we are taught to forgive others and to not hold grudges. This is both for our well-being and theirs.

CHAPTER 3:
Scared Right Out of My Chair

THERE WAS A TIME in my life when I thought post-secondary education was beyond my reach. It's a harrowing ordeal for disabled persons to overcome living in a world built for able-bodied people with minimal to no assistance or awareness. For me, as a Black, disabled Muslim, thoughts of failure and disappointment tend to overshadow my hopes and dreams 90 percent of the time. The other 10 percent is used up putting other individuals' needs before my own—which is the opposite of narcissism—where my sense of self-gratification lies in the excessive interest of catering to other's mindsets.

Leading up to this point, you may be thinking, "Hey, Abdi is a really positive guy"—and I am— which is where the term AbdiPositivity comes from. It actually started off as a joke in 2018, when I was twenty-two. I was playing video games with my buddy Luke, and I'm not sure what we were talking about but it must have been something positive because AbdiPositivity popped in my head, and I have been using it ever since. And although by its very name it is a positive thing, I have unfortunately also used the term as a bargain to lock physical (and some emotional) trauma out of my head. Why? Because though I'm very grateful for my life, AbdiPositivity allows me to have a normal outlook on things, where I am distracted from my very own, often-painful reality. What I didn't know was that my potential was locked inside me, and it was just waiting for the door to be opened. All I needed to do was find the key in myself. If that meant struggling to get into a few doors before that, based on the size of my wheelchair, then so be it. At the end of the day, finding my own happiness was something that I was determined to do, no matter what the outcome and obstacles would be.

Now I wake up with a smile every day and thank God for all of my blessings. I try to find a positive in every scenario in my life, and I look at the glass as half-full rather than half-empty. I acknowledge that some days are harder mentally and physically than others, but there are twenty-four hours in a day, and if I don't smile, then it is left unfulfilled.

Some of the things I have attempted have had good outcomes, and some not so much, but the most important lesson is that I've learned from them. In life, you live and you learn. And if you don't learn from those moments, then how is any journey in life going to become more impactful? So, take a deep breath, get all the jitters out, and ready, set, go. And, remember it's not a race, it's a marathon. Also, make sure to smell the roses, and I mean that literally and figuratively. There's nothing better than smelling a few roses to make your day even more blessed.

CHAPTER 4:

18 Going on Positivity

IN 2014, TOWARD THE end of my final high school semester, I signed up for Youth at Work, a four-week summer program that provides people with disabilities a paid opportunity to work in the community.

For the first two weeks, I worked at Holland Bloorview Kids Rehabilitation Hospital—which in addition to being a rehabilitation centre, is also a school for students with mental or physical disabilities that offers customized hands-on assistance— writing for their official magazine *Bloom*. I used to go there as a student from kindergarten to grade one, so pursuing the program only made sense. It fit my accessibility needs and did not feel like an obligation in any manner. Holland Bloorview was also a safe space for me because I knew the ins and outs of the place very well.

With *Bloom*, I was given the opportunity to write my personal story for my article. I shared my journey of becoming a young adult and going through struggles—both physical and emotional. Crafting my tale was not something I was prepared for, but it was actually pretty fun to let my guard down and just be myself. It was an amazing feeling, and quite frankly, liberating.

The last two weeks, I worked at the campus radio station The Scope at Ryerson University, now known as Toronto Metropolitan University. This is where I had my first genuine exposure to working in the radio broadcasting industry, and I was more than ready to get my hands dirty, so to speak. I was ready to immerse myself in all that was radio. I will never forget the first time I recorded a commercial for the station. I was scared right out of my chair. I say that because I never really saw myself as someone who was capable of working in the community, let alone the broadcasting industry, which can be very competitive and overwhelming. Radio broadcasting includes being exposed to the public, asking myself questions like "Will they like my voice," and the nerves that come with being heard by many people. I thought that people would not accept me for my true self. That is why hiding behind a microphone allowed me to forget my fear of being judged by preconceived notions of what a person like me can or cannot do and instead, I just let my personality shine. It actually had a positive effect on me, when it could have made me too scared to try. After all, in the studio, I was the only one aware of my reality.

Thinking about that time, I do have lots of regrets. I definitely could have humbled myself a bit more instead of 'rolling' away from my personal insecurities. I wanted things to go my way, and if they didn't, I would stay focused on that one issue and make it bigger. Once I was late for my placement, and I forgot to call in to let them know I was running behind. I was worried about getting there so it had slipped my mind. I took this situation and dwelled on it for hours on end. I vividly remember not enjoying working for a bit because I was constantly stressing about the little things like this. My buddy Casey really calmed me down and was able to knock some sense into me though. He said some encouraging and comforting things, like: "Don't worry," "It'll be okay," and "Make sure to breathe." After that, I think I was able to finally enjoy the many great moments I had during my co-op there. For instance, Casey and I co-wrote a fun blog for the radio station's website talking about our experiences as people with disabilities. By the end of the placement, I knew I would want to return in some capacity if I were welcome.

Youth at Work was a big opportunity for me to build the foundation for my professional future. Ironically, it almost didn't happen because I did not initially apply for that program; I originally applied for The Independence Program (TIP) at Holland Bloorview, a summer program run at the University of Toronto, where people with disabilities are given the opportunity to live on their own. For instance, you buy your own groceries, cook your own food (with some assistance), and are responsible for directing your own care, things like telling the personal support workers to come at the times that you prefer. However, I did not get in, as I did not meet the age requirements. Despite this, I strongly believe that not getting the opportunity at TIP was one of the biggest blessings to ever happen to me because instead, the interviewer offered me a position to be a part of Youth at Work. During this period, I started to come to the realization that my dreams were slowly but surely lining up the way they were supposed to. At that point in my life, I was willing to do anything to seize the moment, starting with my placement at Youth at Work.

In October 2014, just three months after I completed my Youth at Work placement, I was invited back to The Scope as a volunteer. I had the privilege of hosting my own thirty-minute pre-recorded show called *Music with Abdi*. Going in, being my first time as a radio-show host, I thought it was going to be the easiest thing in the world. Boy, was I wrong! I had a hard time reading the script and being able to pronounce some of the artists names and songs, so Luke Williams, my technical producer, aided me in reading and pronunciations.

It was such a rush to hear my voice on the radio, and it was a very fulfilling, almost surreal experience. I remained a volunteer at The Scope until April 2016 and it was a special time I will never forget

CHAPTER 5:

Luke

WHEN THE STAFF AT The Scope appointed Luke as my technical producer, he was hosting his own show at the station. I was a bit hesitant about the prospect of working with Luke (nothing against him), mostly because I was imagining the worst before the ball really started to get rolling. I thought Luke would intimidate me, because he was already in university and had much more experience than me in the field of broadcasting. My mind was always programmed to believe the worst before anything ever happened. Back then, I thought this was a good thing, but today, I realize it is terrible. Now I try to look at the positive in any scenario before the negative, and I recommend that others try to do the same, no matter what life throws at you.

The rest, as they say, is history. Luke and I got close, and he became a big part of my life after our time at The Scope. We have shared so many amazing memories together. To give you some perspective of how close we have become, a few years ago my wheelchair broke down while we were at an event together. Now you can probably imagine how freaked out and embarrassed I was to have that happen to me in a public setting, but Luke adapted to the situation in the most beautiful way... so much so that I was awestruck. He was so calm and managed to make me laugh in the midst of my internal chaos. Luke pushed my exceedingly heavy chair, manually, and was willing to come with me all the way home. But instead, we went over to his house to play video games and have pizza, which was our original plan. I was also able to meet his wonderful fiancé at the time, and now wife, Laura. In the past, people would overreact, which would cause me to become stiff and frustrated, making the matter worse than it already was. But Luke was different. I think that was the exact moment I realized that he was going to be a brother for life.

I strongly believe that Luke and I deserve our very own Netflix series titled: *Welcome to the World of Abdi and Luke: A Story of Two Best Friends But More Like Brothers, Trying to Navigate the Craziness of the Twenty-First Century That may Include Me Crashing* into *People and Eating an A&W Burger with Onion Rings*. I have a feeling it would be bigger than *Tiger King*, *Love is Blind*, *Grey's Anatomy,* or *Breaking Bad*. Brian Cranston and Ellen Pompeo would probably be jealous of us. Jokes aside, Luke is a big inspiration to me because he is the first person to make me feel like my disability does not define me.

Luke and I go to sporting events like the Canadian Football League to watch the Toronto Argonauts play the Hamilton Tigercats (Luke lives in Hamilton, so I always dread hearing him brag about the Tigercats because I am an Argonauts fan).

I also helped him with his CBC documentary about gaming accessibility. This was something he was really proud of accomplishing, and I'm thankful that I was with him during the process.

I remember one specific moment when we were actually recording something for the documentary. I believe he said he had tears in his eyes because of the excitement he saw in my face while we were playing video games. Side note—in the years that I've known him, that's the only time I've seen him cry. I'm glad I was able to bring a sense of joy to him, and it is now part of our brotherhood, and something I will never forget. We've always had goofy times together, but to experience that moment filled with raw emotions was very gratifying, to say the least. I hope we have more of those types of experiences together in the future.

To be honest, I am not much of a gamer. Not because I don't like playing, but because there was never much of an accessibility component back then. When Microsoft finally came out with something suitable to my needs, in terms of gaming, I finally felt included. The buttons were much bigger and easier to navigate. To be able to enjoy doing this with one of my best friends was just the icing on top of the cake.

But I think the most important thing I have had the privilege of being part of with Luke, is witnessing him get married in 2019. Going to the wedding dinner was really heartwarming. To support one of my best friends on the happiest day of his life brought me to tears and simultaneously brought me hope that I will get married one day too. I don't know when and where our next adventure will be, but I know it is going to be one for the record books.

If I keep talking about Luke I will just boost his ego, so look out for us in Hollywood, or maybe even in outer space. Let's just say, there is never a dull moment with us.

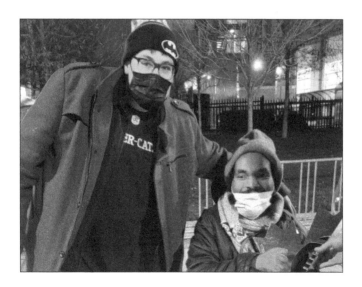

CHAPTER 6:

A Future for the Taking

GOING BACK TO SEPTEMBER 2014 (before I got my volunteer position at The Scope), I contacted a team of post-secondary planners, with an objective of discovering which programs would be suitable for a guy like me. Initially, I spoke to them about a career in journalism because in high school, my goal was to potentially work in media, so I could show off my ever-captivating, George Clooney-level, handsome face to the world— that's a joke... or is it? Despite this long-held ambition, there was something telling me that radio broadcasting was my true calling. This is because I love to talk, and I love having meaningful conversations with people.

Once I had decided on pursuing studies in radio broadcasting, I wanted to be the first physically disabled person to have his own national radio show, so I could show the world who the real Abdi Hassan was, beyond the person in the wheelchair. I guess, in my mind, having my own radio show would have been a dream come true because not only was I aiming to encourage others with the same challenges as me to pursue their dreams and aspirations, but I was also trying to prove that anything is possible if you set your mind to it.

While I was sure of what I wanted to do in life, as I got older, I realized that the transitional process of moving from an isolated environment to the real world would involve facing some of the biggest obstacles I ever had. For instance, being at home for two years straight after three years of going to school every day was something that my mind was used to, but I was not ready for what was to come. I say this because until the COVID-19 pandemic started back in 2020, most of us did not truly understand the affect that seclusion can have on us, especially considering social interaction is such a big component of our humanity. After being at home isolated for two years during the pandemic, it then became difficult to adjust my mind to face life outside of that.

Because of this fear of moving into the real world too fast, I decided to take a year off after graduating high school, which was a big relief because I wanted to explore my options and start branching out in order to find my independence. I continued my volunteer duties at The Scope, while also going out and making more connections with new people in the city. On a few occasions, I went back and visited my old high school, reminiscing about that chapter of my life that had recently come to an end. With a little bit of guidance, I knew I could things on my own.

CHAPTER 7:

Rolling into College Life

IN SEPTEMBER 2016, I continued my journey, and enrolled in the Broadcasting – Radio diploma program at Seneca College. Being the negative Nancy that I was, I started making assumptions about the challenges I was going to face in college. Were my classmates going to accept me for who I was? Would they be comfortable around me? Were all my accessibility needs going to be met? Thankfully, once I got there, I quickly realized I had nothing to worry about. All of my classmates over-looked my challenges, and they treated me the way I always wanted to be treated—equally and fairly, just like everyone else.

Navigating campus alone was new territory for me. I was used to being around a lot of supportive staff members in high school and elementary—ones who always had some form of control over my independence. Nevertheless, I knew that like any new challenge that came my way, I was going to find my way through it. One of the things that helped me was knowing that God was always with me.

One of the first people I met at Seneca College was radio veteran, professor, and program coordinator, Jim Carr. Jim was a wonderful support to me throughout September 2016 until April 2019. He was like the cool uncle that you wanted to brag about to your friends—and he was one of the first teachers, ever, that I didn't try to run over with my wheelchair (surprising, I know). No word of a lie, I think Jim is why I was able to graduate the program with honours. Either that or the old Abdi charm finally paid off.

To this day, I still consider Jim as a father figure in my life. He was always very honest with me, even when I really didn't want to hear it. He treated me just like everyone else in the program, and that is all I had ever wanted throughout my years in the school system. I had finally been given the respect I deserved as a human being.

For the record, when Jim decides to retire as the coordinator of Seneca's Broadcasting – Radio diploma program, I would be honoured to take over his role and continue shining a bright light in the world of media for more people like me.

The broadcasting industry has changed over the years, from when families would gather around the only 'wireless' in a home to listen to an old-time radio program, to now listening to programs from around the world on satellite radio from your phone. You never know, maybe one day somebody will broadcast a radio show from outer space, playing songs like "Fly Me to the Moon" by Frank Sinatra or "Can't Help Falling in Love" by Elvis Presley. Maybe it will be me. Needless to say, the possibilities are endless in the world of broadcasting, especially for people with physical and mental challenges, whether that is behind the mic or in front of the camera. Now back to my story.

Overall, every single person in my program made a huge difference in my life, and I cannot thank them enough for that. Michael, Adam, Connor, Mario, and Dylan, who are my best friends and family, played a key role in my success at Seneca.

Dylan helped me produce a lot of commercials that I had to present in class, and he acted as my second voice. I just love being around him, and he was so patient with me while I was recording, always giving me good suggestions to make my projects stand out more.

Dylan is also a talented musician who has the ability, in my opinion, to sell out Madison Square Garden, singing alongside John Mayer, if given the opportunity.

My buddy Adam is literally the kindest soul I have ever met. Every time I am around him in any capacity my heart is filled with joy. I think one of my favourite memories together was when I did a radio documentary for one of my classes about my journey through adulthood living with a disability. I had to interview a few people and one of the individuals that I selected was Adam. I remember I had my phone recorder on and we were just talking like we normally do, so I almost forgot that I was working on a documentary. I think we spoke for more than an hour and everything just felt organic and peaceful during the entire process. Adam is the man. We've always had this ongoing joke that he and I could be co-sexiest men alive. I'm not sure why that is something that always makes us laugh. In some instances, I want to make it a reality. So *People* magazine... we are waiting for your call.

Michael is one of the most determined and dedicated individuals I know. He always made sure to look out for others in our program, and any time anyone had an issue that needed attention, they went to him. When I was sick for two weeks during my second semester and had to stay home, I had a lot of assignments to catch up on. For three Fridays straight, Michael and I went to the campus, booked a studio, and he helped me work on any projects that I was missing. He basically became my go-to guy during the program. Afterwards, we would go out to eat and Michael would take the time to feed me, even though he didn't have to. That was very heartwarming, and I thank him for everything he has done for me. Michael is multi-talented and what the future holds for him is beyond his very own expectations. I can genuinely say the same for everyone mentioned in this chapter.

Connor was probably the first person I gravitated toward when I first began the radio program. His infectious laughter, self-awareness, and outpouring of love and support for me always put a smile on my face. My favourite memory with him, hands-down, actually happened once we both left the program. We decided to finally go out to dinner after we had been planning it for years while in school. I remember that sunny fall day vividly because my body was so stiff, and I was discouraged and embarrassed of my situation in that moment. But once we sat down at the restaurant, all my worries just went away. His simple presence was able to block all of those negative emotions out. At home the next day, I decided to record a video/thank you letter, which I later posted to social media, dedicated to Connor about what that special day meant to me. FYI, he gives the best hugs, so if you need a hug from Connor let me know... just kidding.

My friend Mario, aka the captain, and I are a lot alike. We are both huge sports fans, specifically of the Toronto Raptors and professional wrestling, but I think what really makes us so connected is that we are both so passionate about our work. Mario is also like my Dr. Phil/Oprah. I speak to him over the phone every week, and I always somehow find myself complaining about something, in a good way.

When I first started writing my book, every time I called him for a year, he would ask me, "How is the book coming along?" At times, I thought he was more passionate about the project than I was, and for crying out loud, I was the one who was writing it. But that meant the world to me and I would not change our friendship for the world. By the time I'm done writing this chapter, I will probably call him again and complain about something, once again in a good way. I am surprised he hasn't charged me for all the times I complain to him.

A description that I believe fits each of their respective characters is that they are all down-to-earth and compassionate people who would move mountains for those they care about. Luckily for me, I just happened to fall in that category.

Moreover, my educational assistants Kim and Brian, along with my friend Fayth, had more hands-on roles in my college success, besides my classmates and professors. They helped me with scribing my notes in class and test/exam preparation.

Let's start with Kim. She was the first EA I had in college. I have worked with many educational assistants over the years, and Kim was probably the best. Her teaching style and the way she made me think while putting my assignments together was unmatched. I am truly grateful for her. Unfortunately, I only got a chance to work with her for one semester, but her impact really shaped the rest of my time at Seneca College. She really set the bar for my success.

Brian, aka brother Brian, and I first met when he became my scribe in first semester. A scribe is someone who helps anyone with physical or mental challenges complete their exams. When I first met him, I could tell we were going to hit it off. Just like Mario, Brian and I are also huge basketball fans. As a Raptors fan, I loved that after I completed my final exams, for about twenty minutes straight, we talked about his love of the New York Knicks and how disgusted he was with them—trust me they were embarrassing to watch in 2016. Brian is someone I have so much love and respect for. When I asked him if I could mention his name in the book, he was very honoured, as if I am a celebrity like JK Rowling. I hope he doesn't pass out once I give him his autographed copy.

Fayth was my technical producer when I was doing my radio show on campus. Her energy is out of this world. Her passion for mental health advocacy is something that makes me so happy to see.

During my last year, she literally became my go-to person, helping me with my assignments and radio show. My classmates that I began the program with graduated in 2018, but I was doing an extra year because I had dropped a total of four courses in my first and second semesters, and I had to make them up. So, the only person I really relied on was Fayth. As the people I knew left, she was the main person

I knew and turned to during that extra year. I felt so bad because she had so much on her plate at the time, but we worked really well together. I always say this, but I do not believe I would have graduated without her help. She acted as my educational assistant, my technical producer, and my good friend, which is more important than anything. I hope I made you proud, Fayth.

Without all these people, I probably would not have finished school. I am grateful for every one of them.

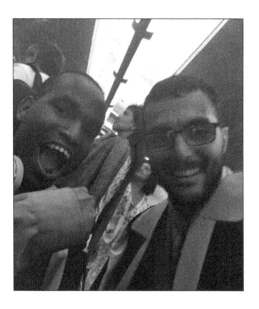

CHAPTER 8:

A Diploma Later

THE DAY I FINALLY graduated the Broadcasting – Radio diploma program on Saturday, June 22, 2019, was the most exhilarating moment of my life. All the blood, sweat, and tears I put into my work had finally paid off. I have never looked forward to anything more than my convocation ceremony.

When I drove across the stage—without crashing into the dean of Seneca College and all the other dignitaries—and received my diploma, it felt like I was the king of the world. I think some of this exuberance and lack of nerves came from the fact that the Toronto Raptors had just won their first NBA championship just nine days prior.

Of course, to commemorate the occasion, I had to take a selfie with the GOAT himself, Jim Carr. Knowing that I was going to be a part of his legendary photo album of graduates was an honour in itself. Jim has been such a big inspiration to me and pivotal to my success. Once again, thank you, Jim. Once my memoir is released, dinner is on me.

A cool moment while I was driving up on stage was when Mario, who also graduated that day with me, was yelling from the top of his lungs in excitement. Everything came full circle for the two of us that day. Mario and I started the program together, then received our diplomas together, a year later than most of our peers because Mario, like me, had to make up a few extra courses. If you want to call it fate, then call it fate. I couldn't have wished for anything more, knowing that I came into my journey as an apprentice, and I left a professional.

Hitting this important milestone in my life, supported by people I cared about, was a feeling like no other. If I had the chance to relive it, I would... a thousand times over. A memorable moment with my mother was when she bought me a blue blazer that I wore to graduation day with my gown. She was at the ceremony and so was my older brother Mohammed and my younger sister Hamdi. It meant a lot to me that my family attended, and I will forever cherish the memory of that day.

Full disclosure, once I graduated the program, I felt lost for a little bit. I had a good feeling that I was going to get a job in the industry right away, but that wasn't the case. So I tried to build my own pathway. I started a weekly blog called "Motivational Talk with Abdi," where I released a motivational blog every Monday for about six months straight. I treated it very seriously, like a paid job, almost like I was working for the *Toronto Star* or the *Globe and Mail.*

As time progressed, the global pandemic hit, I lost my father, which I talk about in the next chapter, and so many other little things were on my plate. But I still kept on doing what I was doing. I continued releasing blogs, and I also started "The AbdiPositivity Podcast," using this as a way to start building the AbdiPositivity brand. Of course, there were a lot of ups and downs, but the radio broadcasting teachers helped me to think outside of just working in the industry and to be able to carve my own path, and the program opened doors beyond my wildest dreams.

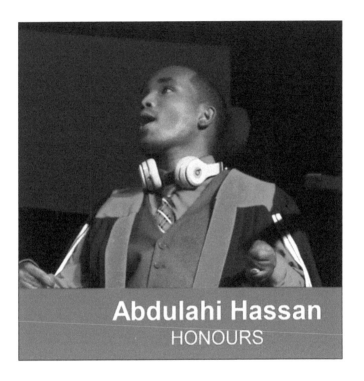

CHAPTER 9:

The Process of Grief

ONE OF THE HARDEST days of my life was the day my father Hussein passed away from an unexpected and sudden stroke. His death was a complete shock to me. He was my better half, and simply put, he completed me.

By the grace of God, I know we will see each other again. I know he would be very proud of me for continuing to honour his legacy every single day that I live on this earth.

I remember my father walking into my room one quiet Sunday night for a routine check-in. He asked me if I needed anything, and I said I didn't. He proceeded to sit on a chair beside me; my television was on in the background, making soft noise. I recall being on my phone the entire time, and I never really struck up a conversation with him. Just a couple of days later, he had a stroke. He was in the hospital for about ten days before he eventually passed away on June 20, 2020. I ask myself every day, "Why didn't I put my phone down?" and "Why didn't I spend the time talking to him?" That Sunday night still weighs heavily on me, and I will always regret my actions. If I had the chance to relive that evening, I would put my phone down and spend every moment with him.

I have so many fantastic memories with my dad... of him being in the hospital with me when I had surgery on my legs, and then simply being at home and hanging out, just the two of us, once or twice a week for the last ten years.

Sometimes we did things individually, but we would still keep each other company. Other times we would watch wrestling, basketball, or anything that brought us close together. My father would use words that are not appropriate to express his love of professional wrestling and when watching basketball with me. He'd jokingly say, "Why am I always supporting the Raptors? Do I get paid to do it?"

Let's just say that the Raptors gave us a lot of stress as a family, especially during playoff times.

My father once said that I was not human. Let me share the backstory to this statement. We had guests over from the United States in the summer of 2013, and I wanted to get out of bed and onto my chair, so my father and my cousin Abdifitah were going to lift me. In that moment, my dad just said the first thing that came to his mind, and that was me not being human. I know it isn't true, but it still makes me laugh.

I will be honest that I used to be a little selfish and was not patient with him. I would lash out on him at times for no apparent reason. I blame that on my ego and some personal issues. May God forgive me for those actions.

Seeing what an incredible parent my father was, I made a promise to myself that if I am ever to have any children, God willing, I will bestow my father's name, Hussein, upon a son—and a daughter will be named Halimo, after my father's sister, who passed away years ago.

Full disclosure, Aunt Halimo was my favourite aunt. She was one of the funniest and most caring people I have ever known. Sorry to my siblings when you read this, but she would call my dad once a day, and the only two people she would ask about was her brother and myself. One memory I have of her is when I needed to use the washroom and we had multiple guests over the night, for whatever reason, and I remember I needed to go so badly that I was screaming at the top of my lungs for somebody to help me, but no one came. My aunt Halimo, who wasn't capable of assisting me to the other room, was crying her eyes out because nobody was there to help me. Long story short, my other aunt came to save the day.

I miss my dad and my aunt very much, but I know I will see them both again someday in the afterlife, God willing.

Nobody is ever prepared to lose a loved one, but it is a reality of life. Every soul alive will taste death, but the shock and grief I felt after losing my father is something that I still feel deeply. I do take comfort in thinking that he is in a better place and not suffering.

At the end of the day, I just have to continue moving forward because I know that is what my dad would want for me. He will always be remembered in my heart as the greatest dad in the world, my first real best friend, and a person who loved me more than I could ever love myself. Sometimes, when I am alone in my room, I feel like he is there, having a conversation with me and letting me know everything will be okay, but I know deep down, that it is Allah reassuring me. I believe my father would want me to pray for him and also to speak up for myself since his voice is no longer there for me.

The funeral and time of mourning was incredibly painful, however, special at the same time. I had the opportunity to see many of my family members—some who I had not seen since I was a kid. Having family and cousins there added a beautiful light in that time of darkness. I talk about this almost all the time, and it is really one of those moments I wish I could relive. So many family members came by my house after the funeral, and I remember that I was just lying down on my bed as floods of people came in and out of my room, almost like a hotel suite. They offered me and my family their condolences and that simple gesture really warmed my heart.

To be honest, after a while I just wanted to be alone and grieve peacefully, but then I remembered that my cousins Sofia and Nasra, who prior to the funeral, I had not seen since 2017—or maybe even longer than that—were coming to visit. I thought because of their busy schedules and personal lives they were only going to be around for a few minutes (and I would have been more than okay with that), but they ended up staying for more than an hour with me. Just to see them both was more of a treat than anything else. It truly meant so much to me that they did that. I have had so many tremendous conversations in my lifetime but hands down the one I had with the two of them tops them all. It felt very raw, emotional, and authentic. I think it was one of the few times in my life that I was able to let my guard down and convince myself that it is okay to be vulnerable instead of being very guarded and scared of showing real emotion. I was simply true and human.

As I said, I hope to honour my dad every single day and take care of all my family members, especially my mom, who has been the strongest individual in my life; going through the process of grief, while getting used to the dynamic of being the head of the house and taking care of me and my siblings. I think over the last two years, we have gotten closer than ever. It's funny because my mom never leaves the house without saying goodbye to me and vice-versa. That has become our own little ritual. I have the best mom in the world, and I always envisioned that I would be able to buy her a house of her own.

Life is so unpredictable; so much so that after grief and loss, it still goes on like nothing happened. This idea of a continuously smooth journey is so weird to me because when you lose someone you really care about—who has taken care of you since your first breath—your whole world comes to a standstill. So, to push through, for the sake of my own sanity and my father's honour, I kept a positive mindset by doing motivational blogs, posts, quotes, and as I mentioned earlier, starting my own podcast titled The AbdiPositivity Podcast. All of these things have kept me going, knowing I have people who depend on me to give them the motivation to start their day right, as well as my late father's expectations of me that I want to uphold to honour his memory.

Despite everything, I appreciate the good times as well as the bad because without those moments, I wouldn't be who I am today. Even though he will never get a chance to read my book, I know that I will meet him again and read it to him myself. My dad is my biggest inspiration to writing this memoir. The process of grief was the first chapter I wrote in the beginning of this whole experience and is the one I keep coming back to.

This chapter specifically has put me through a rollercoaster of emotions, to say the least. I'm grateful for the lessons that grief has taught me along the way, like it's okay to let your guard down, if you need to cry, cry, and if you need to laugh based on a memory, go ahead and do it. Allow yourself to express who you are, and that includes the good, the bad, the ugly, the funny, etc. As I mentioned before, grief is strange. And surprisingly, I'm strangely happy that we have grief as a tool of emotion that can be expressed in different forms. For me, that was writing this chapter.

So, my advice to anyone who is dealing with any form of grief, is to fight it rigorously. You are not alone. There will always be a shining light waiting for you. In the Holy Quran, God says "Verily, with hardship comes ease." Yes, if I'm being honest, I still struggle with my dad not being here. But time heals all. Every day I feel something different, but I always remember that I'm moving forward not backwards, even while dealing with grief. I just have to not lose faith in myself or God, go with the flow, and conquer every day like it is my last. It is also mentioned in Islam that when a loved passes away, the best thing you can do is remember them and the best form of remembering them is by praying for them. And that's what I will continue to do until my last breath on this earth. I love you, dad.

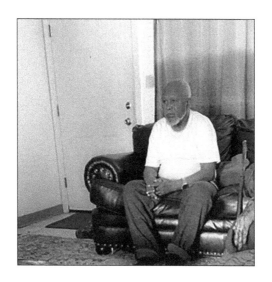

CHAPTER 10:

Finding Happiness While Dealing with Grief

AS I HAVE SAID, grief is the most unpredictable concept that any human will deal with in their lifetime. But I have also come to realize that there is a happy side of grief. You might be thinking… how does that work? Well, I'll tell you. A couple of years ago, I was on a Muslim dating app, and I came across a profile of a girl who will remain nameless for the sake of privacy. I was feeling good, so I said to myself, "Let me do something spontaneous and send her a message." One of the first things I said to her was, "I don't have any ill intentions," and I asked her what her purpose in life was. I sent the message, then went back to watching television, wrestling to be exact. In the back of my mind, I thought she would not answer and that would be the end of it. Five minutes later a notification popped up on my phone, and it was from none other than herself. My first reaction was shock, with butterflies in my stomach. She responded better than I expected. We proceeded to text for two hours straight, about anything and everything.

I will be honest; I was definitely going through a dark period in my life during that time. I was still grieving the loss of my father. But every time I spoke to her, it felt like an escape from my reality. Over time my feelings for her grew into something, but I couldn't exactly describe what those feelings were. Even though she came into my life at a time where things were very uncertain, I didn't want to lose her. She was my happy place in the midst of grief. So, when she disappeared for a few months from social media, that being our only source of communication, it was heartbreaking. Every time I bragged about her to my peers and family, I would smile like I had never smiled before. She was the first person that I barely knew that left a huge impact in my life. I will always pray for her and ask

God that if she is meant to be in my life, then let her be. But if not, then I'll be happy with the outcome and be grateful regardless for every moment I had with her. A lot of my peers said to be careful because they were looking out for my well-being, and I love and respect them for that. However, I knew that she was meant to be in my life for one reason or another. Like I said, whenever she would disappear off of social media, I knew that she would be back in some capacity.

It is safe to say that as time went on, I fell in love with her, but I was too scared to admit it. I used my disability as a coping mechanism to avoid *speaking my truth*. Every time I would attempt to make connections with people or try to pursue something in the romance department, I would get scared to enter that new territory. My fear of getting heartbroken and judged by others stopped me from taking risks and going beyond my limits. This individual has taken all of those fears away.

Even though she might not realize it, maybe she was put in my life for a reason. I guess time will tell. I underestimated how much the little things meant to me, especially when you are describing your love for someone. For instance, every time I posted something on social media and she liked it, it made my heart smile. It felt like every worry in my life went away. Each time we connected, in any form, whether having conversations or interacting through posts, I said to myself, "This is something that I can't take for granted and whatever comes out of the situation, I'll be happy." Even if I don't get a chance to tell this to her face to face, hopefully she will read it through my memoir. This whole thing has taught me that it is okay to express your deepest emotions rather than bottling them up. This results in having a big weight lifted off of your shoulder, along with clarity and a peace of mind.

CHAPTER 11:

My Message for the World

I'VE TALKED ABOUT MANY personal things in my memoir, like the passing of my father, falling in love, and fears about attending college. Obviously, no one knows what the future holds for anyone. I think that's an interesting dynamic because people are so focused on what's going to happen tomorrow that they forget to live in the moment. I can admit that I've struggled with that for years because I never thought I'd be able to build a future. I trained my mind to believe that the concept of having aspirations didn't exist. But once I was in college, I started to believe that I could build a future. I want to get married, I want to have kids, and I want to establish my AbdiPositivity brand as a motivational speaker. By the will of God, it will happen. I want to give people a sense of hope—hope that I should have given myself.

Now, we all know as humans that tomorrow is never promised. But my message to anyone reading this is to not waste your life. Dwelling in the past can hinder your potential and believe me, I know that struggle. One thing that helped me take negative thoughts out of my head was being able to accept and love myself, including the flaws and challenges that I deal with. We all create our reality with our thoughts, so it is important to keep a positive mindset and conquer our biggest obstacles, turning them into our biggest successes. And if life gets too hard, just take a breath and tell yourself how great you are, with a smile on the side.

Obviously, some days are going to be more difficult than others, but never forget that every individual has control of his/her narrative. At the end of the day, the chapters in your life won't be authentic if you don't direct your narrative. Yes, people might tell you what to do and where to go, but its ultimately up to you how your journey will end. You will have bumps along on the road, and you will experience new things. You will come across people in your life that make you ask yourself, "Why are they here?" But it goes back to what I reiterated at the beginning: life is unpredictable. But the beauty that comes in those moments will hopefully give you a brighter perspective on your future, but more importantly, you as an individual. Try to find gratitude in every adversity that comes your way because that's the foundation of building great character. That is one of the best feelings in the world. So, stay humble, stay grateful, be kind to yourself and others, make sure to tell those around you that you love them, and give yourself a pat on the back for all that you've accomplished; even if it's from helping yourself or others.

CHAPTER 12:

Never Say Never in the World of Abdi

AFTER MANY MONTHS OF discussions with friends and family—not to mention lots of prayer—I finally decided to write my memoir. As the saying goes, time waits for no one. Writing this book is one of the greatest achievements of my life, besides graduating college, posting motivational videos/ quotes, and writing blogs, etc. There were times where I doubted myself and wondered if I should do it. In February 2021, before I opened the Word document and begin dictating, I called my friend Conner and told him that I wanted to start the project but had concerns that were holding me back. I recall him saying, "Just write and have fun doing it." In that moment, I knew he was right. So I turned off my phone, said a quick prayer, and began writing like there was no tomorrow. I will admit that at times, I would not allow myself to take a break. Once my mind is set on something, I refuse to slow down. This is something I know a lot of people can relate to. When you are passionate about something, it feels like it's just you against the world. Sometimes we can be our own worst enemies, and it will be hard to comprehend that.

Nonetheless, I was ready to take the journey and whatever came with it—the good, the bad, the ugly, the complicated, the not-so complicated, and everything in between.

I didn't just get up one morning and say to myself, "Hey, I need to write a book and become a *New York Times* best-selling author." First, I drove around my hallway, crashed into a few walls, got a Big Mac combo from McDonald's, and then came to the realization that I wanted to write a book about my life. Finding the courage to tell my story is something that I am extremely proud of.

I can't even tell you how many times I doubted my ability to do this, but the process was made much easier by praying about it, as well as talking to Connor, Mario, and my family. I could focus on all the things that I can't do, but I choose to focus on what I can do, and what I hope others do as well. I just want people to read my story and be motivated to do better and be the best that they can be. Once again, time waits for no one. Eventually our time on this earth will come to an end, and I just want people to feel like they can achieve anything they set their mind to, no matter what limits there may be. We are only as good as we make ourselves out to be.

This is also a thank you letter to any family members, friends, classmates, professors, or anyone I had a brief encounter with (whatever the case may be), thank you... because without those moments, this book wouldn't have been possible. Wherever my journey takes me next, I just hope to smile like nobody is watching (and eat lots of good food, preferably a Subway steak and cheese sandwich, an M&M cookie, and a can of Pepsi). I know that I am diabetic, but even reminiscing about a Philly cheesesteak from time to time is such a beautiful feeling that can't be described.

Writing my memoir for over a year has given me so much hope for my future. When I started, I forgot to have fun with it, and I treated the process like a nine to five job, worrying about the little things, which is something I now know I would have done differently. Looking back, it has been one of the biggest blessings in my life, and I would do it all over in a heartbeat. I surprisingly would want to relive all the emotions again, including the stressful times, heartache, and the "what-ifs." "Trust your process" was the saying I lived by during this entire journey. Every scenario I went through while completing this project was a part of the process. I just hope to continue growing each day, inspire the people around me (regardless of what struggles I deal with on a daily basis), laugh in times of uncertainty and, most importantly, reach out to God every chance that I get.

Eventually I know that time is going to stop. It's inevitable. I hope after I'm long-gone people will remember me as a person who brought them joy, even if we only came across each other once. I've met many great people in my lifetime, and some of them have told me how inspirational I am. What they don't know is that I get that inspiration from many different people from all walks of life. Even though I do appreciate them saying it, I am just a human who has unique challenges and tries to live a normal life, while attempting to make others happy in the process. Because, as they say, sharing is caring, and happiness is a universal shared emotion that deserves to be spread around.

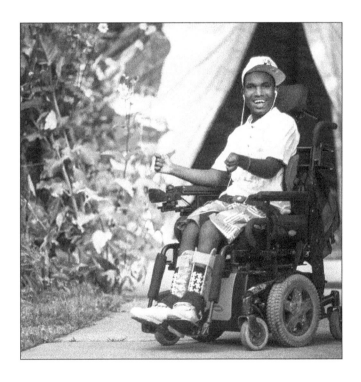

CPSIA information can be obtained
at www.ICGtesting.com
Printed in the USA
LVHW071912270223
740524LV00049B/2504

9 781039 158900